Amani Ben Mansour
Henda Neji

Infectious lung disease: interest of the CT

Amani Ben Mansour
Henda Neji

Infectious lung disease: interest of the CT

Management of patients hospitalized for infectious pneumonia: interest of the thoracic CT scan

ScienciaScripts

Imprint

Any brand names and product names mentioned in this book are subject to trademark, brand or patent protection and are trademarks or registered trademarks of their respective holders. The use of brand names, product names, common names, trade names, product descriptions etc. even without a particular marking in this work is in no way to be construed to mean that such names may be regarded as unrestricted in respect of trademark and brand protection legislation and could thus be used by anyone.

Cover image: www.ingimage.com

This book is a translation from the original published under ISBN 978-620-3-44546-6.

Publisher:
Sciencia Scripts
is a trademark of
Dodo Books Indian Ocean Ltd. and OmniScriptum S.R.L publishing group

120 High Road, East Finchley, London, N2 9ED, United Kingdom
Str. Armeneasca 28/1, office 1, Chisinau MD-2012, Republic of Moldova, Europe
Printed at: see last page
ISBN: 978-620-5-55059-5

TABLE OF CONTENTS

INTRODUCTION

Acute community-acquired pneumonia (CAP) is an acute infection of the lung parenchyma acquired outside the hospital or within the first 48 hours of hospitalization or more than 14 days after a hospital stay[1,2].

Its incidence varies between 1.7 and 11.6 per 1000 inhabitants per year [3]. It is considered a public health problem because of its frequency and morbidity, thus contributing considerably to the expenses of the health care system. Indeed, it represents the first cause of mortality by infectious disease in Western countries [1]. In Europe, 2.3% of annual deaths are due to CAP. Mortality varies widely depending on the place of care and can reach 40% in intensive care units (ICUs) [2].

The definition of CAP is radio-clinical [4,5].Bacterial evidence of infectiony is infrequent and late. The diagnosis is based on the association of general and respiratory signs of infection with radiological involvement. Almost a third of patients have no signs, hence the importance of imaging [4,6].

Imaging is based primarily on the frontal chest X-ray, which is recommended by the various scientific societies; however, there are limitations to this examination, including the presence of grey areas and poor agreement between radiologists, radiologists and clinicians, and between clinicians.

Computed tomography (CT) seems to be a good alternative. However, its place in patients with a confirmed diagnosis remains poorly defined and less well documented.

The objective of our work was to evaluate the diagnostic contribution of thoracic CT and its impact on the therapeutic management of patients hospitalized for CAP.

METHODS

1. Type of study

This is a retrospective descriptive study conducted over the period fromJanuary 2015 to March 2019 and collating patients hospitalized for CAP in Pavilion C of AbderrahmanMami Hospital of Ariana and explored by thoracic CT or thoracic angio-CT.

2. Patients

2.1. Inclusion criteria

Included in this study were patients:

- with CAP diagnosed on the basis of clinical and radiological signs.

- who had a thoracic CT or thoracic CT-angiogram

- over 18 years of age

2.2. Non-inclusion criteria

Patients were not included:

-with acute bronchitis, bronchial obstructive pulmonary disease (COPD), bronchial dilatation infection or pulmonary tuberculosis in any form.

- not hospitalized, whose management was strictly ambulatory.

2.3. Exclusion Criteria

- Patients whose medical records were incomplete and did not allow for adequate data collection were excluded.

3. Methodology

3.1. Data collection

The medical record was the primary source of information.

We collected data, from hospitalization records including:

- Epidemiological characteristics (age, sex, smoking habits, especially smoking in pack years (PA), cardiovascular history, especially diabetes, respiratory history: COPD, asthma, renal failure, cancer ...).
- Functional signs (dry cough, productive cough, exertional dyspnea, chest pain, hemoptysis, fever, asthenia, myalgia)

- Clinical examination data on admission (respiratory rate, heart rate, blood pressure, cardiopulmonary auscultation, peripheral oxygen saturation)
- Biological data (white blood cell count, neutrophil count, sedimentation rate, CRP, renal assessment)
- Bacteriological data (sputum cytobacteriological examination, blood cultures, pneumococcal and legionella antigenuria, atypical serologies)
- Arterial gasometry
- The specific severity score for pneumopathy: CURB 65 score (Appendix 1)
- Chest X-ray data: Non-systematized alveolar opacity, acute lobar frank pneumonia, interstitial syndrome, bilateral opacities (bronchopneumonia), excavation, localization of abnormalities, presence or absence of pleural syndrome and/or mediastinal silhouette anomalies.
- Thoracic CT data: indication, technique (examination with or without contrast injection, thoracic CT angiography, time to request from admission, results).
- Therapeutic management: initial therapeutic management and after the result of the CT scan

3.2. Ethical considerations

3.2.1. Patient safety

This is a retrospective, observational, non-interventional study.

3.2.2. Security of personal data

The security of patients' personal data was respected and guaranteed. The databases used for the statistics were anonymous.

3.3. Method of statistical analysis of results

For categorical variables, we calculated simple and relative frequencies (percentages).

For the quantitative variables, we calculated the means and determined the extreme values.

3.4. Bibliographic research

-Search engines: PubMed, Google Scholar, Cochrane, ClinicalKey.

-Sites: ScienceDirect, Masson.

-Research limitations: the last ten years

RESULTS

1. Epidemiology and general characteristics of the population

One hundred and eighteen patients were hospitalized for CAP during the study period, of whom 41 patients had chest CT scans. Nine patients were excluded for missing data. A total of 32 patients were included in this study.

1.1. Age

The average age of our patients was 60.2 ± 14.5 years with extremes ranging from 23 to 84 years.

1.2. Type

Our study included 21 male patients (65.6%) and 11 female patients (34.4%)

1.3. Habits and pathological history

Active smoking was found in 20 patients (62.5%). The average smoking rate was 28 PA.

The most frequent respiratory history was chronic obstructive pulmonary disease in 11 patients (34.3%), asthma in 4 patients (12.5%) and severe obstructive sleep apnea syndrome in one patient.

The most noted cardiovascular comorbidities were arterial hypertension in 7 cases (21.9%), diabetes in 4 cases (12.5%), and arrhythmia in one case.

 A history of moderate renal failure was noted in one patient (3.1%).

A history of CAP was noted in 3 patients: right in two patients

and left in a patient.

2. Clinical parameters at admission

2.1. Functional signs

The onset of symptoms was progressive in 50% of patients with a mean time between the onset of symptoms and consultation of 11.5 days.

The most frequent reasons for consultation were fever in 21 cases (65.6%), productive cough in 14 cases (43.8%), asthenia and chills in 10 cases each (31.3%), dyspnea in 9 cases (28.1%), dry cough, chest pain, hemoptysis in 7 cases (21.9%) each, myalgia in 6 cases (18.8%) and arthralgia in 2 cases (6.3%).

2.2. Clinical signs

Fever was present in 19 patients (59.3%). A respiratory rate higher than 20 cycles/min was found in 12 patients (37.5%). The examination showed the presence of signs of struggle in 21 patients (65.6%).

On pulmonary auscultation, condensation syndrome was present in only 10 patients (31.2%).

Table I summarizes the vital parameters found on admission examination.

Table n° I Vital parameters of patients at admission

Parameter	Median Per [25-75]
Respiratory rate (cycles/min)	22 [15-32]
Heart rate (bpm)	100 [66-132]
Systolic blood pressure (cmHg)	12 [10-16]
Diastolic blood pressure (cmHg)	7,5 [6-10]
Peripheral Oxygen Saturation (%)	88 [79-94]

2.3. Reasons for hospitalization

The reasons for hospitalization in our series were acute respiratory failure in 23 cases (71.8%), decompensation of associated defects in 5 cases (15.6%), failure of home management in 2 cases (6.25%), unfavorable socioeconomic conditions in one case (3.1%) and predictable therapeutic noncompliance in one patient (3.1%)

3. Additional examinations

3.1. Biology

On admission, 16 patients (50%) had a leukocytosis ≥ 10,000 elements/mm3. Anemia was found in 9 patients (28.1%) including 3 men and 6 women. Twenty patients (62.5%) had a CRP greater than 5 mg/dl.

Table II summarizes the values of the biological parameters studied at admission.

Table n° II Biological parameters of patients at admission

	Median Per [25-75]
Urea (mmol/L)	8 [4-16]
Creatinine (µmol/L)	63,5 [44-123]
CRP (mg/L)	86 [22-331]
Leukocytes (10^3 e/mm^3)	11780 [9400-17500]
Hemoglobin (g/dL)	11,5 [8,5-15]
Platelets (10^3 e/mm^3)	175 [122-321]

3.2. Microbiology

Sputum cytobacteriological examination (SCC) was performed in 25 patients (78.1%). It was contributory in 5 patients.

The bacteriological workup isolated the causative germ in 6 patients (18.75%). Streptococcus pneumoniae was the most frequently isolated germ

(4 patients). In addition, Klebsiellepneumoniae was involved in one case (3.1%) and Legionellapneumophila in one case (3.1%).

4. Initial severity score CURB 65

The majority of patients (37.5%) had a CURB-65 of 1. Figure 1 shows the distribution of patients according to severity as assessed by CURB-65.

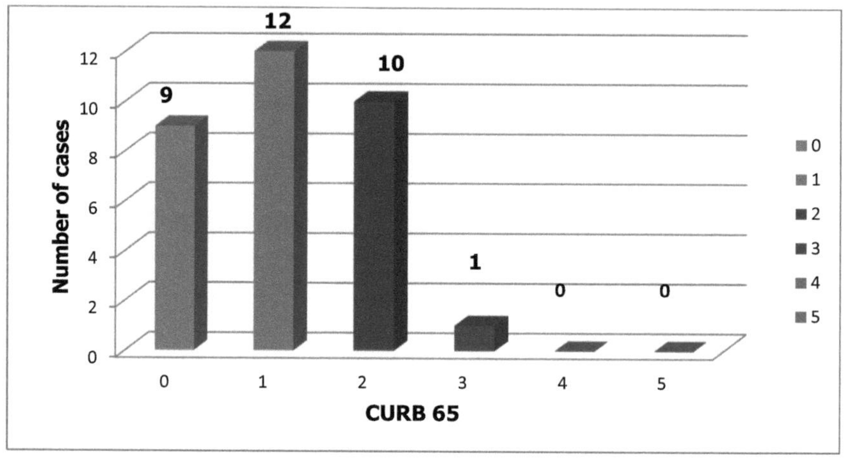

Figure 1: Distribution of patients by CURB-65

5. Chest X-ray

All patients had a chest X-ray on admission.

The most frequently observed radiological abnormality was an unsystematized alveolar opacity in 16 patients (50%) (Figure 2). In addition, there was an appearance of acute lobar frank pneumonia in 5 cases (15.6%) (Figure 3), bilateral opacities suggestive of broncho-pneumonia in 8 cases (25%) (Figure 4) or interstitial syndrome in 4 cases (12.5%). Excavations were present in 4 cases (12.5%).

The abnormalities were essentially unilateral, most frequently located on the right (14 patients or 43.7%).Table III summarizes the radiological aspects and distribution of the lesions.

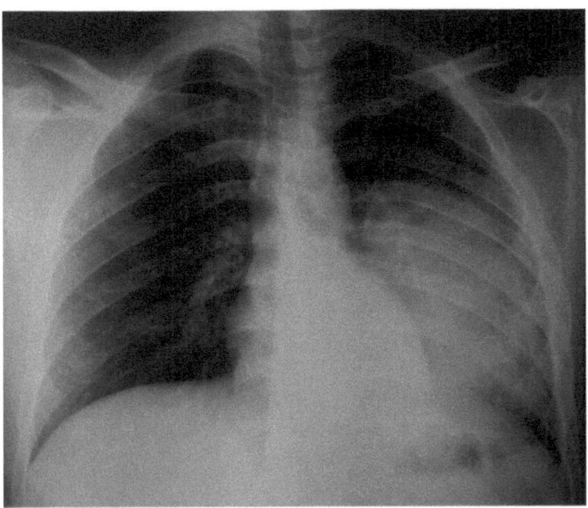

Figure 2: Frontal chest radiograph of a patient admitted for CAP showing nonsystematized alveolar opacity not obliterating the left border of the heart of inferior lobar seat.

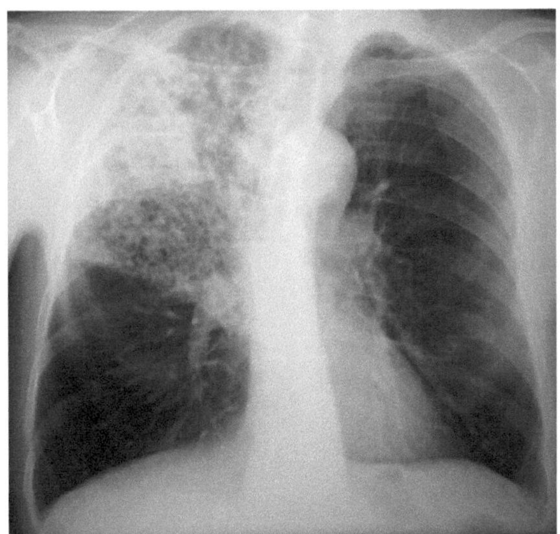

Figure 3: Frontal chest radiograph of a patient submitted for CAP: heterogeneous, systematized right upper lobar alveolar opacity

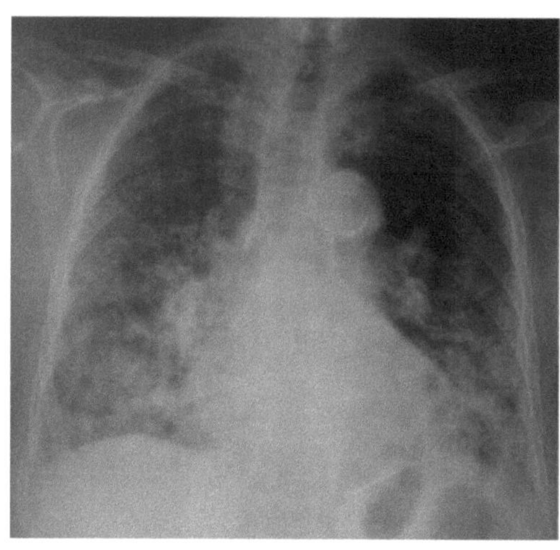

Figure 4: Frontal chest radiograph of a patient admitted for CAP showing bilateral alveolar opacities suggesting bronchopneumonia.

Table n° III Aspects and distribution of radiological lesions in our series

Anomalies	N (%)
non-systematized alveolar opacity	16 (50)
Appearance of acute lobar frank pneumonia	5 (15,6)
Interstitial syndrome	4 (12,5)
Bilateral opacities	8 (25)
Excavation	4 (12,5)
Left location	11 (34,4)
Location right	14 (43,7)
Associated pleural syndrome	2 (6,3)
Anomalies of the mediastinal silhouette	0

6. Initial therapeutic course of action

In our series, an initial probabilistic antibiotic therapy was started in all patients. The choice of the antibiotic family was made according to the clinical, radiological and bacteriological orientation.

Monotherapy was initiated in 25 patients (78.1%). Dual therapy was prescribed in 7 patients (21.8%). Amoxicillin/clavulanic acid was the most prescribed antibiotic as monotherapy in 22 patients (68.7%), followed by Cefotaxime and Levofloxacin.

Other measures associated with antibiotics were: oxygen therapy in 21 patients (65.6%), non-invasive ventilation in 3 patients (9.3%), bronchial drainage physiotherapy in 29 patients (90.6%) and short-acting Beta2 mimetics in 5 patients (15.6%).

7. Thoracic CT scan

Chest CT scans were performed in all patients.

7.1. Technique

This was a thoracic CT scan without iodinated contrast injection in 7 cases (21.9%), a thoracic CT scan with contrast injection in 7 cases (21.9%) or a thoracic angioscan at the pulmonary artery time in 18 cases (56.2%).

7.2. Time to request a chest CT scan

The mean time to request a chest CT scan from the date of admission was 2.6 days ± 1.08 days.

7.3. Indications

The indications of the thoracic CT in our series were

- Suspicion of pulmonary embolism in the majority of cases: 18 cases (56.3%) (6 patients had a high clinical probability score (revised Geneva score) and 12 patients had an intermediate clinical probability score.

-lack of response to prescribed treatments in 14 patients (43.8%)

- aggravation of the infectious syndrome in 8 cases (25%)

- radiological aggravation in 4 cases (12.5%): noted on average after 72 hours of hospitalization. It was the extension of the alveolar syndrome in 3 cases (Figure 5) and labilateralization of the lesions in 1 case

- the appearance of a hydroaerobic level in 3 cases (9.4%) (Figure 6)

- the appearance of a pleural opacity under treatment in 2 cases (6.3%)

- the guidance of a possible thoracic drainage in 3 cases (9.4%).

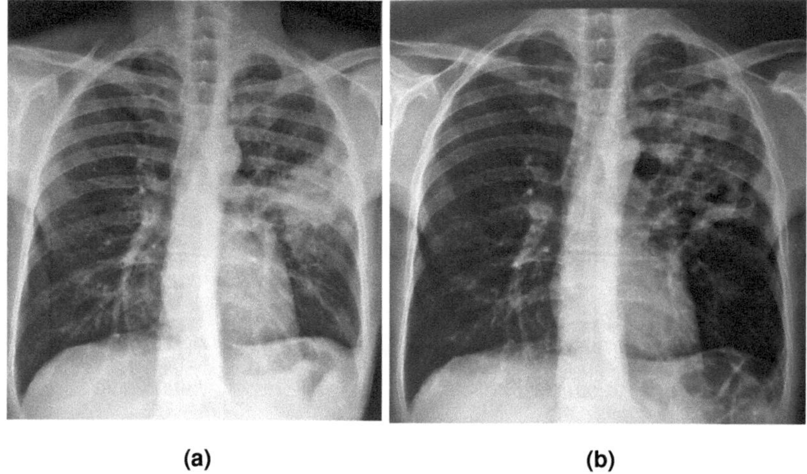

(a) **(b)**

Figure 5: Chest radiographs of a patient treated for CAP. **(a)** Chest radiograph on admission: left hilo-axillary alveolar opacity with blunting of the left pleural cul de sac. **(b)** Radiograph at H48: worsening with extension of the left alveolar opacity and appearance of excavations

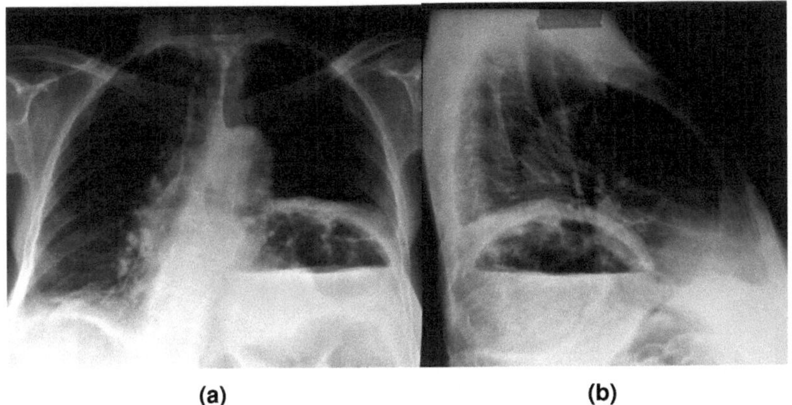

(a)   **(b)**

Figure 6: Chest radiographs of a patient treated for CAP after 24 hours of hospitalization (a) frontal radiograph: rounded opacity of the lower 1/3 of the left lung field excavated with a hydro-aerial level horizontally (b) profile radiograph: constant appearance of the hydro-aerial level suggestive of a pulmonary abscess

7.4. Results of the thoracic CT scan

Among the 18 patients who had a thoracic angiography scan, the diagnosis of pulmonary embolism was confirmed in 5 patients (27.8%) and invalidated in the remaining 13 patients (72.2%).

These were proximal right pulmonary artery thrombosis in 1 case (Figure 7), distal right thrombosis in 3 cases and bilateral pulmonary thrombosis in 1 case.

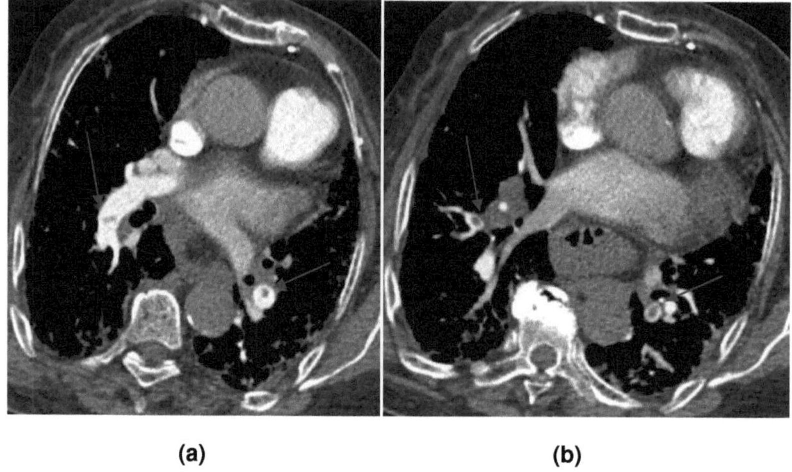

(a)   **(b)**

Figure 7: Chest CT angiogram of a patient admitted for CAP, requested at H 48. (a and b) Mediastinal window sections showing bilateral pulmonary artery thrombosis.

-In the group of patients in whom a pulmonary embolism was invalidated, the chest CT scan further showed:

* localized bronchial dilatation with signs of superinfection in 6 patients (18.7%),

* parenchymal descondensations in 5 patients (15.6%) which were bilateral associated with bronchiolar micronodules in 2 of them (Figure 8).

* cellular bronchiolitis in 2 patients (6.25%).

-In the group of patients not improved on antibiotic treatment, the chest CT scan objectified:

* elementary lesions of diffuse infiltrative pneumonitis whose appearance and distribution were suggestive of PHS or PINS in one patient (3.1%),

* a large necrotic tissue mass with pleural invasion and signs of carcinomatous lymphangitis in a patient

*excavated parenchymal condensations in 3 patients (Figure 9)

* associated ventilatory disorders in 2 patients (6.25%): partially ventilated collapse in one patient and atelectasis by rolling in the other.

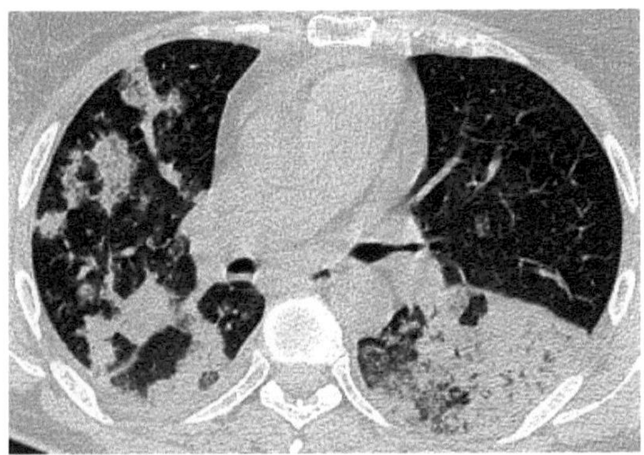

Figure 8: Axial section in parenchymal window showing bilateral parenchymal condensations associated with areas of ground glass hyperdensity suggestive of bronchopneumonia.

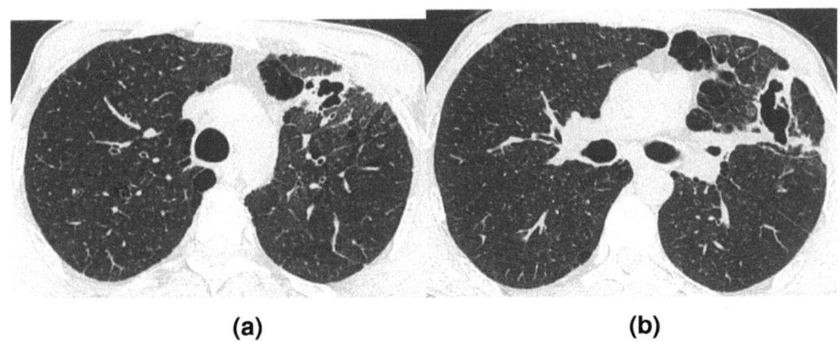

(a)   (b)

Figure 9: Parenchymal window axial sections of a patient admitted for CAP on D2 of hospitalization, showing the presence of multi-excavated parenchymal condensations of the culmen

-In the group of patients in whom we noted the appearance of a hydroaerobic level, the thoracic CT scan showed an aspect of pulmonary abscess in 2 cases (6.25%) (Figure 10), and an abscessed pneumopathy ruptured in the pleura in one case (3.1%).

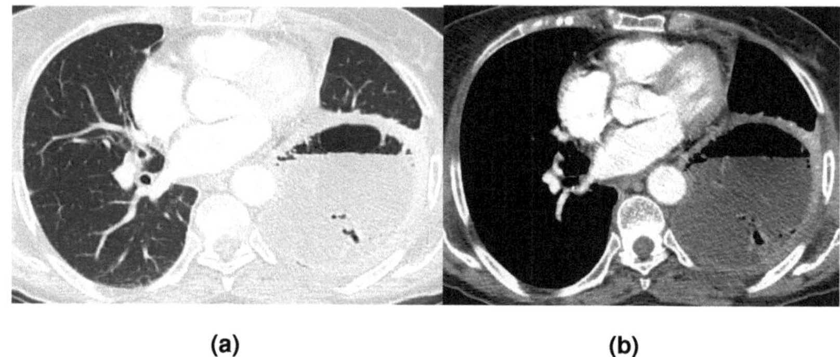

(a)   **(b)**

Figure 10: Chest CT scan of a patient admitted for left-sided CAP with the appearance after 24 hours of hospitalization of a hydro-aerated level.

(a) (a) axial section in parenchymal window and (b) axial section in mediastinal window: large multi-walled fluid collection in the left lower lobar with a hydroaerobic level having an acute angle of connection with the thoracic wall, suggestive of a pulmonary abscess

-In the group of patients in whom a worsening of the infectious syndrome was objectified, the thoracic CT scan showed an aspect of abscessed pneumopathy in one patient (3.1%) and an encysted pleural effusion in one patient (3.1%).

Table IV summarizes the different findings of the chest CT in our series.

Table n° IV Summary table of the results of the thoracic scanner

Result	N (%)
Confirmed pulmonary embolism	5 (15,6)
Localized bronchial dilatation with signs of superinfection	6 (18,7)
Parenchymal condensations	
• excavated	3 (9,3)
• localized	4 (12,5)
• bilateral	2 (6,25)
Cellular Bronchiolitis	3 (9,3)
Lung abscess	3 (9,3)
• complicated by rupture in the pleura	1 (3,1)
Ventilation disorders	2 (6,25)
• partially ventilated collapse	1 (3,1)
• Coil atelectasis	1 (3,1)
Necrotic tissue mass with pleural invasion and signs of carcinomatous lymphangitis	1 (3,1)
Encysted pleural effusion	1 (3,1)
Pleural thickening associated with pleural leaflet enhancement and low-level pleural effusion	1 (3,1)
PID whose appearance and distribution are suggestive of PHS or PINS	1 (3,1)
Signs of chronic lung disease	1 (3,1)

7.5. Impact of chest CT findings on therapeutic management

A change in antibiotic therapy was initiated after the result of the CT scan in 5 patients (15.6%). A macrolide was added in 2 cases (6.25%) when the CT scan revealed bilateral involvement. The spectrum of antibiotic therapy was extended in 3 cases (12.5%) in the presence of pneumopathy complicated by abscesses.

Antibiotic therapy was discontinued in 2 patients (6.25%): one patient with a CT scan showing signs of COPD without any other scan sign suggestive of a focus of lung disease, and one patient with a proximal pulmonary embolism without a focus of lung disease.

Curative anticoagulant therapy was initiated in 5 patients (15.6%) with confirmed pulmonary embolism.

Intravenous corticosteroid therapy was added to one patient, who was diagnosed with acute hypersensitivity pneumonitis (HSP) on CT data.

DISCUSSION

CAP is the leading cause of morbidity and mortality from infectious diseases, making it a public health problem [2].

The diagnosis is based on clinical and biological findings. Chest X-ray is the only radiological examination for diagnostic purposes that is recommended in the first instance. CT is usually indicated in cases of clinico-radiographic discordance. Its place in patients with a confirmed diagnosis at initial presentation remains poorly defined and less well documented.

We performed a retrospective evaluation of the indications, outcomes, and therapeutic impact of CT scanning in patients hospitalized in Ward C with the diagnosis of CAP. We collected 32 patients during the period from January 2015 to March 2019. The mean age was 60.2 ± 14.5 years with a sex ratio of 21/11. CT was performed without iodinated contrast injection in 7 cases and with contrast injection in 7 cases (21.8%). Thoracic CT angiography was indicated in 18 patients. The average time between hospitalization and the request for a thoracic CT scan was 2.6 days. The indications were mainly suspicion of pulmonary embolism in 18 cases (56.2%), lack of response to the prescribed treatment in 14 cases (43.7%), worsening of the infectious syndrome in 8 cases (25%), radiological worsening in 4 cases (12.5%), appearance of a hydro-aerosic level in 3 cases (9.4%) and guidance for a possible thoracic drainage in 3 cases (9.4%). The diagnosis of pulmonary embolism was confirmed in 5 patients (27.8%). In addition, the thoracic CT scan showed the presence of localized bronchial dilatations with signs of superinfection in 6 patients (18.7%), parenchymal condensations in 5 patients (15.6%) which were bilateral associated with bronchiolar micronodules in 2 patients, the presence of excavated parenchymal condensations in 3 patients, a pulmonary abscess appearance in 2 patients (6.25%), and an abscessed lung disease ruptured in the pleura in one patient (3.1%).

A change in antibiotic therapy was imposed by the results of the thoracic CT scan in 5 patients (15.6%). Antibiotic therapy was stopped in 2 patients (6.25%). Anticoagulant therapy at curative dose was instituted in 5 patients (15.6%).

Intravenous corticosteroid therapy was added in one patient.

The strength of our work is that it evaluates a diagnostic procedure and its therapeutic impact. We have shown that the thoracic scanner has allowed a modification of the therapeutic behaviour in more than a third of the patients (13/32 patients). However, our work has the limitations of any retrospective study, especially concerning data collection. The 2ème limitation is the sample size. Moreover, the study only included patients from ward C and would not reflect the diagnostic attitude in the whole hospital.

1. Diagnosis of acute community acquired pneumonia

The diagnosis of CAP is difficult. It is based on a combination of clinical and radiological findings. The clinical and radiological data are dependent on the examination technique and the experience of the examiner. Clinical signs are rarely complete. The use of an en face chest radiograph is recommended as soon as the diagnosis is suggested. The risks of diagnostic error are 2-fold:

- the risk of overdiagnosis of CAP when an opacity of non-infectious origin coexists with fever [7]: bronchoceles, pleural sequelae, bronchial cancer, pulmonary infarction, atelectasis, organized pneumonia, pulmonary edema, vasculitis... [8].

- the risk of not recognizing a PAC when the constitution of the opacity is late compared to the clinic. Indeed, 2 to 7% of early stage CAPs have a normal chest radiograph [9]. The difficulties of radiological diagnosis are maximal in the elderly because of the frequent prior existence of pulmonary parenchymal abnormalities of respiratory or cardiac origin, the high prevalence of bronchopneumonia and the difficulty of performing chest radiography in non-cooperative patients. [10]. The injection-free CT scan has its place in these difficult situations. The angioscan is reserved for the elimination of a pulmonary embolism.

2. Epidemiological characteristics of patients

Our patient population is marked by an advanced age with an average of over 60 years. Indeed, the prevalence of CAP is increasing in this age group. In France, it is estimated between 400,000 and 600,000 cases/year [11]. In Tunisia, there are no precise figures for the incidence of CAP in the elderly. The increased susceptibility of the elderly to respiratory infections is explained by the anatomical and physiological changes of the respiratory system related to aging [12]. In addition, other age-independent risk factors are comorbidities, smoking, alcoholism and socioeconomic status.

In our series, COPD was the most frequent respiratory comorbidity. In the literature, the most frequent comorbidities favoring CAP are COPD, chronic heart failure and diabetes [1]. These comorbidities are taken into account in the severity scores. They have a specific weight in the prognosis of CAP [1]. This was confirmed in the multicenter (including ten centers), longitudinal, prospective study of Fernandez-Fabrellas et al [13] comparing the characteristics of patients with CAP according to the coexistence or not of COPD, whether the patients were managed in hospital or as outpatients. The analysis included 1,282 CAP patients, 906 without COPD and 376 with COPD. The group with COPD was older and had more comorbidities, but there was no difference in radiological characteristics or extension of the lung disease. The COPD group developed acute respiratory failure more often (20.7% versus 11.3%, p<0.001), but were not admitted to an intensive care unit more often.

3. Clinical evaluation

The clinical signs (functional and physical examination) that can lead to the diagnosis of CAP are very numerous. In our population, the most noted clinical signs were productive cough in 14 cases (43.8%), asthenia and chills in 10 cases each (31.3%), dyspnea in 9 cases (28.1%), dry cough and chest pain in 7 cases (21.9%) each, hemoptysis in 7 cases (21.9%), myalgia in 6 cases (18.8%). Fever was present in 19 patients (59.3%). The examination showed the presence of signs of struggle in 21 (65.6%) of the patients. On pulmonary auscultation, condensation syndrome was present in only 10 patients (31.2%).

Our results are similar to those of other studies. Indeed, the signs most frequently found during CAP are cough, dyspnea, latero-thoracic pain, sputum, fever, tachycardia, polypnea, global impression of severity, localized dullness and crepitus focus [13].

Some signs have a higher value, such as the presence of crepitus in lateral decubitus persisting on inspiration [14].

Based on the clinical elements, and in order to rationalize management, it has been suggested that a set of signs could define CAP. Thus, it could correspond to a picture whose semiology would be based on the association of a temperature greater than or equal to 38°C associated with more than one of the following acute respiratory signs: cough, sputum, dyspnea, chest pain, change in pulmonary auscultation. This consensus definition is used by investigators to include homogeneous patient populations in studies, including impact or high-level evidence studies. However, there is a lack of clinical sensitivity particularly in the elderly patient. Signs that are inconsistent in the young adult are even more inconsistent in the older patient [14].

4. Place of the thoracic radiography

In our series, all patients had a chest X-ray on admission. Indeed, the use of a chest X-ray is mandatory as soon as the diagnosis is evoked. In case of a normal initial X-ray, a control of the face will be carried out if the clinical suspicion persists [1].

CAPs are manifested by opacities of very diverse appearance. In our series, the most frequently observed radiological abnormality was a non-systematized alveolar opacity in half of the cases. In addition, 5 cases (15.6%) had an acute lobar frank pneumonia appearance, a quarter had bilateral opacities suggestive of broncho-pneumonia, and 4 cases (12.5%) had an interstitial syndrome. Excavations were present in 4 cases (12.5%).

Our results are in agreement with data from a Tunisian study performed in 2015 at the Abderrahmen Mami Hospital in ariana, evaluating the clinical features of CAP in the elderly, where the most frequently found radiological appearance was a non-systematized alveolar opacity [14]. **On the** other hand, these opacities may evolve towards systematization, with or without air bronchogram. This aspect is the most easily recognized and most frequently reported in severe forms [1,7].

Chest radiography in CAP also has its place during surveillance. In our series, radiological aggravation was documented in 4 cases (12.5%) and was noted on average after 48 hours of hospitalization.

Indeed, the absence of clinical response, in particular of fever defervescence, 48 to 72 hours after the start of treatment, is an indication to repeat the chest radiograph, looking for a complication, or an argument for the verification of the initial diagnosis [1]. **During the course of the disease,** the persistence of clinical symptoms or auscultatory abnormalities beyond the usual time of resolution is an indication to repeat the chest radiograph [1].

Thus, the latter compensates for the relative insufficiency of functional signs and physical examination. Nevertheless, the interpretation of chest radiography remains a controversial issue. Several authors have demonstrated that there is interobserver heterogeneity in the interpretation of these radiographs **[6]**. Albaum et al. conducted a study on 282 chest radiographs (Table V) which showed that, on the same image, two radiologists frequently have conflicting interpretations **[6]**.

Table no. V Concordance between 2 radiologists regarding the diagnosis of CAP **[6]**.

Question asked	Answers provided	Agreement on the answers	Kappa
Infiltrate	Yes	79,4 %	0,37 (0,22-0,52)
	No	6 %	
Distribution	Unilobar	41,50 %	0,51 (0,28-0,62)
	Multi-lobed	33,90 %	
Pleuresis	Yes	10,70 %	0,46 (0,33-0,50)
	No	73,20 %	
Character	Alveolar	93,60 %	- 0.01 (- 0,03 - 0,00)
	Interstitial	100 %	
Air Bronchogram	Yes	7,60 %	0,01 (- 0,13-0,15)
	No	52,90 %	

5. Place of the thoracic scanner

5.1. Time to request a chest CT scan

The mean time from hospitalization to the request for a chest CT scan in our series was 2.6 days. This is explained by the recommended time for clinical and therapeutic reassessment. Indeed, in outpatient and inpatient settings, a clinical re-evaluation is mandatory at 48-72 hours. It will lead to a modification or maintenance of the antibiotic prescribed in first intention according to the clinical evolution and the relevant microbiological results when they are available **[16]**.

5.2. Indications

In our series, the indications were essentially a suspicion of pulmonary embolism in 18 cases (56.2%), a lack of response to the prescribed treatment in 14 cases

(43.7%), a worsening of the infectious syndrome in 8 cases (25%), a radiological worsening in 4 cases (12.5%), the appearance of a hydro-aerosic level in 3 cases (9.4%) and guidance for a possible thoracic drainage in 3 cases (9.4%)

These results are consistent with the literature. In fact, a chest CT scan is performed if the radiograph is difficult to interpret or if there is no response to the initial treatment to eliminate a pulmonary embolism or a complication such as a pulmonary abscess or pleural empyema **[17]**.

There are very few studies available evaluating the benefit of chest CT in hospitalized adults with pneumonia. A few authors have reported series of patients who received chest CT scans and were diagnosed with CAP. The main study is that reported by Syrjala et al **[18]**. In this study, on a limited group of 47 patients, with a mean age of 51.4 years (extremes 17-78 years), the authors evaluated the value of chest CT in patients suspected of having CAP (19 inpatients, 28 outpatients). A standard chest radiograph and a chest CT scan were performed simultaneously in all 47 patients. The evaluation was performed by 2 independent radiologists. Standard radiography found CAP in 18 cases (38% lung disease), with bilateral abnormalities in 6 cases. Chest CT scan found abnormalities in an additional 8 patients (17% additional lung disease). The prevalence of lung disease in these patients with suspected CAP thus increased from 38.3% to 55.3% after the CT scan, and bilateral involvement from 12.8% to 34%. The lack of follow-up of the patients in this study does not allow us to state with certainty that the opacities thus diagnosed were indeed PAC.

In the absence of data allowing a large-scale evaluation of the diagnostic and therapeutic value of such an examination, even the 2006 consensus conference on the management of lower respiratory infections was unable to decide on the use of a CT scan for the diagnosis of CAP. However, this examination is recommended in case of diagnostic doubt **[1]**.

5.3. Results

In our study, 18 scans out of 32 (56.2%) were thoracic angioscans motivated by a suspicion of pulmonary embolism. The diagnosis of pulmonary embolism was confirmed in 5 patients (27.8%). Pulmonary embolism is a condition that can mimic or be associated with CAP. The latter is itself a risk factor for thromboembolic disease.

Indeed, in addition to their overlapping demographic characteristics, a patient developing pneumonia is more likely to have a pulmonary embolism [19]. In a study conducted in Great Britain, it was shown that 27 to 40% of patients with pneumonia also had a concomitant pulmonary embolism [19,20]. This is consistent with our results showing the presence of pulmonary embolism in 27.8% of patients with a suspected pulmonary embolism diagnosis.

In addition, in our study, the thoracic CT scan showed a pulmonary abscess in 2 cases (6.25%), and an abscessed pneumonia ruptured in the pleura in one case (3.1%). Indeed, abscesses are complications of bacterial pneumonia, which are encountered in particular during infections with necrotizing and anaerobic germs [21]. The CT appearance is that of single or multiple collections, 2 to 6 cm in diameter, showing central hypoattenuation or cavitation in relation to purulent liquefied necrosis, with peripheral enhancement after intravenous injection of contrast medium [21].

The internal wall of the abscesses is most often irregular, with frequent hydro-aerosic levels and adjacent parenchymal condensation in half of the cases. The preferential locations, related to the frequency of inhalation pneumonitis in this setting, are the posterior segments of the right upper and left lower lobes or the upper segments of the lower lobes [21].

Pleural effusions occur in 20-60% of cases of acute bacterial pneumonia. More than 90% of para-pneumonic effusions, without pleural thickening, regress with appropriate antibiotic therapy. In case of empyema, there is pleural thickening of the visceral and parietal layers after injection of contrast medium, with densification of the extrapleural fat. Pleural empyema must be distinguished from pulmonary abscess [21].

5.4. Impact of thoracic CT on therapeutic management

In our series, a modification of antibiotic therapy was imposed by the results of the thoracic CT in 7 patients (21.8%). Antibiotic therapy was stopped in 2 patients (6.25%). Our results are similar to the results of 2 studies.

The first is the prospective multicenter study by Cleassens et al [22], which aimed to determine the diagnostic and therapeutic impact of chest CT in clinical suspicion of CAP. A chest CT scan with standardized interpretation was performed within 4 hours.

The diagnostic certainty of CAP and the therapeutic plans were established by the emergency physician before and after the scan. The final diagnosis of CAP was established at D 28 by a validation committee. Three hundred and nineteen patients were included. The diagnosis was modified by the thoracic CT scan in 187 patients (58.6%, 95% confidence interval [53.2; 64]), and was consistent with the committee's final diagnosis in 73% of cases. Antibiotic treatment was initiated (51 patients) or discontinued (29 patients) following chest CT in 80 patients (25%). The authors concluded that in cases of clinical suspicion of CAP, early chest CT alters the diagnostic probability in 60% of cases, excludes the diagnosis in 30%, and alters the choice of therapy in 20% of cases (Table VI).

Table n°VI: Therapeutic modifications after thoracic CT scan according to the study of Cleassens YE et al **[22]**

	Pre-CT thoracic		Post-chest CT	
Antibiotic treatment	Initiation	n=207 (65%)	Stop	n=29 (9%)
			Setting up	n=51 (16%)
			Class modification	n=70 (22%)
Other treatments			Anti-coagulation (EP)	n=3
			Diuretics (IC)	n=11
Place of care	Admission	n=250 (78%)	Admission	n=249 (78%)
			Changes	n=45 (14%)
			-ambulatory→ admitted	n=22
			-admitted→ ambulatory	n=23

In a second Swiss prospective interventional study, involving patients over 65 years of age, hospitalized in internal medicine and geriatrics conducted in 2016, any patient with clinical suspicion of pneumonia (at least one respiratory symptom and one infectious symptom), treated with antibiotic therapy since the emergency room could be included **[23]**. Patients treated with antibiotics for pneumonia during the previous 6 months were excluded, as well as those who had received antibiotics for more than 48 hours or had had a chest CT scan for another indication. Chest X-ray and low-dose chest CT were performed in all included patients within 72 hours of admission. The likelihood of pneumonia was assessed by the clinician using a 5-point Lickert scale (excluded, low, intermediate, high, certain) before and after the chest CT scan. The primary outcome was represented by the number of diagnoses modified by increase in diagnostic probability or decrease in diagnostic probability. Of 898 patients, 203 were included. Of these, 154 (75.9%) had community-acquired pneumonia, 72 (35.5%) had been hospitalized during the previous 6 months. The median CURB65 score was 2. 30-day mortality was 5.4%. Eighty-five patients (41.9%) had abnormalities on the en face chest radiograph. The probability of the diagnosis of pneumonia was modified after the CT scan in 134 patients (67 had increased probability and 67 had decreased probability). Antibiotic therapy was discontinued in 18 patients (9%) after the scan. At the end of these results, the authors of this study concluded that the value of the CT scan in the diagnosis and management of these patients lies in particular in the decrease in the use of probabilistic antibiotic therapy.

Thus, the thoracic CT improves management. If it allows to specify the diagnosis, in particular in patients for whom the chest X-ray is less informative and the clinical probability more uncertain, it also allows to modify the management of the patient in a better way. Thus, in the ESCAPED study **[24]**, the performance of a chest CT scan modified the therapeutic attitude in 61% of patients, including antibiotic therapy (discontinuation, initiation, modification), the addition of other specific treatments, and the place of treatment (admission or outpatient). Regarding antibiotic therapy, these modifications allowed a better adherence to the recommendations of good practice for clinicians.

CONCLUSIONS

Acute community-acquired pneumonia (CAP) is a public health problem. It is one of the most common, deadly and costly illnesses and one of the most common indications for hospital admissions.

The diagnosis of these conditions is based on clinico-biological and radiological elements. Chest radiography remains the reference examination recommended at first sight. This rule should not, however, lead to the disregard of certain limitations of this examination, such as the evaluation of the extent of the lesions and their severity, as well as its contribution to the establishment of the etiological diagnosis. These elements can be better studied in CT. However, the role of this examination in patients with a confirmed diagnosis at the initial presentation remains poorly defined and less well documented.

In this context, we conducted a retrospective study, including patients hospitalized in the Pneumology C department of Abderrahman Mami Hospital in Ariana for CAP and explored by thoracic CT or thoracic angiography. The aim of this study was to evaluate the diagnostic contribution of thoracic CT and its impact on their therapeutic management.

We collected 32 patients during the period from January 2015 to March 2019. The mean age was 60.2 ± 14.5 years with a sex ratio of 1.9. All patients had a chest radiograph on admission. The most frequent radiological appearance was a nonsystematic alveolar opacity (16 patients or 50%). The mean time to request a chest CT scan from the date of admission was 2.6 days ± 1.08. The main indication for the CT scan was a suspicion of pulmonary embolism (18 cases or 56.3%). These results are in line with the literature, where this examination is mainly requested in case of diagnostic doubt, allowing to eliminate other differential diagnoses such as pulmonary embolism. The other indications were lack of response to the prescribed treatment (14 patients, i.e. 43.8%), worsening of the infectious syndrome (8 cases, i.e. 25%), radiological worsening (4 cases, i.e. 12.5%), appearance of a hydroaerobic level (3 cases, i.e. 9.4%), appearance of pleural opacity under treatment (2 cases, i.e. 6.3%), and guidance of a possible thoracic drainage (3 cases, i.e. 9.4%) Among the 18 patients who underwent thoracic angiography, the diagnosis of pulmonary embolism was confirmed in 5 patients (27.8%) and invalidated in 13 patients (72.2%). A modification of antibiotic therapy was undertaken after the CT result in 5 patients (15.6%). Antibiotic therapy was stopped in 2 patients (6.25%). Curative anticoagulant therapy was initiated in 5 patients (15.6%). Intravenous corticosteroid therapy was added in one patient.

This result seems to be interesting insofar as it relates the interest of the thoracic scanner in reducing the use of probabilistic antibiotic therapy.

This work has thus contributed to the evaluation of practices in our department. However, some limitations should be noted, particularly the sample size and the retrospective nature of the data collection. Nevertheless, the results of our study could be the first step in the development of other prospective multicenter studies to evaluate the indications and usefulness of chest CT in patients with CAP.

The study of the impact of "low dose" chest CT at the time of hospitalization for CAP could be considered as a first step.

REFERENCES

1. XV Consensus Conference on Anti-Infective Therapeutics, 2006. Management of lower respiratory tract infections in the immunocompetent adult. Medicine and Infectious Diseases, 36:235-244.

2. Gibson GJ, Loddenkemper R, Lundbäck B, Sibille Y. Respiratory health and disease in Europe: the new European Lung White Book. Eur Respir J. 2013 Sep;42(3):559-63.

3. Torres A, Peetermans WE, Viegi G, Blasi F. Risk factors for community-acquired pneumonia in adults in Europe: a literature review. Thorax. 2013 Nov;68(11):1057-65.

4. Moore M, Stuart B, Little P, Smith S, Thompson MJ, Knox K, et al. Predictors of pneumonia in lower respiratory tract infections: 3C prospective cough complication cohort study. Eur Respir J. 2017 Nov 22;50(5):1700434.

5. Blasi F, Mantero M, Santus P, Tarsia P. Understanding the burden of pneumococcal disease in adults. Clin Microbiol Infect. 2012 Oct;18 Suppl 5:7-14.

6. Albaum M, Hill L, Murphy M, Li Y, Fuhrman C, Britton C, et al. Interobserver reliability of the chest radiograph in community-acquired pneumonia. Chest. 1996;110:343-350.

7. Franquet T. Imaging of pneumonia: trends and algorithms. Eur Respir J. 2001 Jul;18(1):196-208

8. Almirall J, Bolibar I, Vidal J, Sauca G, Coll P, Niklasson B, et al. Epidemiology of community-acquired pneumonia in adults: a population-based study. Eur Respir J. 2000 Apr;15(4):757-63.

9. Melbye H, Straume B, Aasebo U, Dale K. Diagnosis of pneumonia in adults in general practice. Relative importance of typical symptoms and abnormal chest signs evaluated against a radiographic reference standard. Scand J Prim Health Care. 1992 Sep;10(3):226-33.

10. Rello J, Rodriguez R, Jubert P, Alvarez B. Severe community-acquired pneumonia in the elderly: epidemiology and prognosis. Study Group for Severe Community-Acquired Pneumonia. Clin Infect Dis. 1996 Oct;23(4):723-8.

11. Jackson ML, Neuzil KM, Thompson WW, Shay DK, Yu O, Hanson CA, et al. The burden of community-acquired pneumonia in seniors: results of a population-based study. Clin Infect Dis. 2004 Dec 1;39(11):1642-50.

12. Hammami S, Chakroun M, Mahjoub S, Bouzouaia N. Infections in the elderly. Rev Tun Infect. 2007;1:1-8.

13. Fernandez-Fabrellas E, Aguar MC, Signes-Costa J, Blanquer J, Sanz F, Martinez-Moragon E, et al. Differences of Community-Acquired Pneumonia in COPD Patients. Am J Respir Critic Care Med. 2007;175:A105

14. Habibech S. Acute community-acquired pneumonia in the elderly: a comparative study [Thesis]. Medicine: Tunis; 2015. 30p.

15. Wipf J.E, Lipsky B.A, Hirsschmann J.V, Boyko E.J, Takasugi J, Peugeot R.L, et al. Diagnosing pneumonia by physical examination: relevant or relic? Arch Intern Med 1999; 159:1082-7.

16. Chidiac C, Ader F. Community-acquired pneumonia in adults. Rev Prat. 2011 Oct;61(8):1077-84.

17. Syrjälä H, Broas M, Suramo I, Ojala A, Lähde S. High-resolution computed tomography for the diagnosis of community-acquired pneumonia. Clin Infect Dis. 1998 Aug;27(2):358-63.

18. Basi SK, Marrie TJ, Huang JQ, Majumdar SR. Patients admitted to hospital with suspected pneumonia and normal chest radiographs: epidemiology, microbiology, and outcomes. Am J Med. 2004 Sep 1;117(5):305-11

19. Kelly J, Hunt BJ, Rudd A, Lewis RR. Pulmonary embolism and pneumonia may be confounded after acute stroke and may co-exist. Ageing. 2002 Jul;31(4):235-9.

20. Goldhaber SZ, Hennekens CH, Evans DA, Newton EC, Godleski JJ. Factors associated with correct antemortem diagnosis of major pulmonary embolism. Am J Med. 1982 Dec;73(6):822-6.

21. Beigelman-Aubry C, Godet C, Caumes E. Lung infections: the radiologist's perspective. Diagn Interv Imaging. 2012 Jun;93(6):431-40.

22. Claessens YE, Debray MP, Tubach F, Brun AL, Rammaert B, Hausfater P, et al. Early Chest Computed Tomography Scan to Assist Diagnosis and Guide Treatment

Decision for Suspected Community-acquired Pneumonia. Am J Respir Crit Care Med. 2015 Oct 15;192(8):974-82.

23. Prendki V, Scheffler M, Garin N, Carballo S, Serratrice C, Marti C, et al. Value of low-dose chest CT in the diagnosis of pneumonia in the elderly. Rev Internal Medicine. June 2017;38:A57- 8.

24. Le Bel J, Pelaccia T, Ray P, Mayaud C, Brun AL, Hausfater P, et al. Impact of emergency physician experience on decision-making in patients with suspected community-acquired pneumonia and undergoing systematic thoracic CT scan. Emerg Med J. 2019 Aug;36(8):485-492.

APPENDIX

Appendix 1. CURB-65 score

Item	Points
Confusion	1
Urea > 7 mmol/L	1
Respiratory rate ≥30 cpm	
Blood pressure	1
Systolic < 90 mmHg	1
or Diastolic ≤ 60 mmHg	1
Age ≥65 years	1

Risk	Points	mortality (%) according to Lim et al.
Low risk	0-1	0,7-2,1
Moderate risk	2	9,2
High risk	3	14,5
Very high risk	≥4	>40

MANAGEMENT OF HOSPITALIZED PATIENTS FOR COMMUNITY-ACQUIRED ACUTE PULMONARY DISEASE: INTEREST OF THORACIC COMPUTED TOMOGRAPHY

Abstract

Background:

Acute community-acquired pneumonia (CAP) in adults is a public health problem with significant morbidity and mortality. Chest X-ray is the first radiological examination recommended to be practiced. Computed tomography (CT) is generally indicated in cases of clinical and radiographic discrepancy. Its place in patients with confirmed diagnosis at the initial presentation remains unclear and less well documented. The purpose of our study was to evaluate the diagnostic contribution of chest CT and its impact on their therapeutic management.

Methods:

Retrospective study, including patients admitted for CAP in the Pulmonology C department of Mami Ariana Hospital from January 2015 to March 2019, and who underwent chest CT or chest CT angiography.

Results:

We enrolled 32 patients admitted for acute CAP. The average age was 60.2 ± 14.5 years with a sex ratio of 21/11. Chest CT was performed without contrast material in 7 cases (21.8%) and with contrast material in 7 cases (21.8%). CT angiography was performed in 18 cases (56.3%). The delay between admission and CT practice was 2.6 days ± 1.08. CT indications included pulmonary embolism suspicion in 18 cases (56.2%), no improvement under treatment in 14 patients (43.7%),infectious syndrome worsening in 8 cases (25%), radiological worsening in 4 cases (12.5%), occurrence of a hydro-aeric level in 3 cases (9.4%) and thoracic drainage guidance in 3 cases (9.4%).The diagnosis of pulmonary embolism was confirmed in 5 patients (27.8%). CT results induced antibiotic therapy modification in 5 cases (15.6%). The antibiotic therapy was stopped in 2 patients (6.25%).

Conclusion:

In patients with CAP, CT allows complications diagnosis, antibiotic guidance and pulmonary embolism confirmation

Key-words : Pneumonia, Thorax , Tomography